I0759081

Table of Contents

How Intermittent Fasting Can Help You Lose Weight

There are many different ways to lose weight.

One strategy that has become popular in recent years is called intermittent fasting.

Intermittent fasting is an eating pattern that involves regular, short-term fasts — or periods of minimal or no food consumption.

Most people understand intermittent fasting as a weight loss intervention. Fasting for short periods of time helps people eat fewer calories, which may result in weight loss over time.

However, intermittent fasting may also help modify risk factors for health conditions like diabetes and cardiovascular disease, such as lowering cholesterol and blood sugar levels.

This article explores everything you need to know about intermittent fasting and weight loss.

Choosing your intermittent fasting plan

There are several different intermittent fasting methods. The most popular ones include:

- the 16:8 method

- the 5:2 diet

- the Warrior diet

- Eat Stop Eat

- alternate-day fasting (ADF)

All methods can be effective, but figuring out which one works best depends on the individual.

To help you choose the method that fits your lifestyle, here's a breakdown of the pros and cons of each.

The 16/8 method

The 16/8 intermittent fasting plan is one of the most popular styles of fasting for weight loss.

The plan restricts food consumption and calorie-containing beverages to a set window of 8 hours per day. It requires abstaining from food for the remaining 16 hours of the day.

While other diets can set strict rules and regulations, the 16/8 method is based on a time-restricted feeding (TRF) model and more flexible.

You can choose any 8-hour window to consume calories.

Some people opt to skip breakfast and fast from noon to 8 p.m., while others avoid eating late and stick to a 9 a.m. to 5 p.m. schedule.

Limiting the number of hours that you can eat during the day may help you lose weight and lower your blood pressure.

Research indicates that time-restricted feeding patterns such as the 16/8 method may prevent hypertension and reduce the amount of food consumed, leading to weight loss.

A 2016 study found that when combined with resistance training, the 16/8 method helped decreased fat mass and maintain muscle mass in male participants.

A more recent study found that the 16/8 method did not impair gains in muscle or strength in women performing resistance training.

While the 16/8 method can easily fit into any lifestyle, some people may find it challenging to avoid eating for 16 hours straight.

Additionally, eating too many snacks or junk food during your 8-hour window can negate the positive effects associated with 16/8 intermittent fasting.

Be sure to eat a balanced diet comprising fruits, vegetables, whole grains, healthy fats, and protein to maximize the potential health benefits of this diet.

The 5:2 method

The 5:2 diet is a straightforward intermittent fasting plan.

Five days per week, you eat normally and don't restrict calories. Then, on the other two days of the week, you reduce your calorie intake to one-quarter of your daily needs.

For someone who regularly consumes 2,000 calories per day, this would mean reducing their calorie intake to just 500 calories per day, two days per week.

According to a 2018 study the 5:2 diet is just as effective as daily calorie restriction for weight loss and blood glucose control among those with type 2 diabetes.

Another study found that the 5:2 diet was just as effective as continuous calorie restriction for both weight loss and the prevention of metabolic diseases like heart disease and diabetes.

The 5:2 diet provides flexibility, as you get to pick which days you fast, and there are no rules regarding what or when to eat on full-calorie days.

That said, it's worth mentioning that eating "normally" on full-calorie days does not give you a free pass to eat whatever you want.

Restricting yourself to just 500 calories per day isn't easy, even if it's only for two days per week. Plus, consuming too few calories may make you feel ill or faint.

The 5:2 diet can be effective, but it's not for everyone. Talk to your doctor to see if the 5:2 diet may be right for you.

Eat Stop Eat

Eat Stop Eat is an unconventional approach to intermittent fasting popularized by Brad Pilon, author of the book "Eat Stop Eat."

This intermittent fasting plan involves identifying one or two non-consecutive days per week during which you abstain from eating, or fast, for a 24-hour period.

During the remaining days of the week, you can eat freely, but it's recommended to eat a well-rounded diet and avoid overconsumption.

The rationale behind a weekly 24-hour fast is that consuming fewer calories will lead to weight loss.

Fasting for up to 24 hours can lead to a metabolic shift that causes your body to use fat as an energy source instead of glucose.

But avoiding food for 24 hours at a time requires a lot of willpower and may lead to binging and overconsumption later on. It may also lead to disordered eating patterns.

More research is needed regarding the Eat Stop Eat diet to determine its potential health benefits and weight loss properties.

Talk to your doctor before trying Eat Stop Eat to see if it may be an effective weight loss solution for you.

Alternate-day fasting

Alternate-day fasting is an intermittent fasting plan with an easy-to-remember structure. On this diet, you fast every other day but can eat whatever you want on the non-fasting days.

Some versions of this diet embrace a "modified" fasting strategy that involves eating around 500 calories on fasting days. However, other versions eliminate calories altogether on fasting days.

Alternate-day fasting has proven weight loss benefits.

A randomized pilot study comparing alternate-day fasting to a daily caloric restriction in adults with obesity found both methods to be equally effective for weight loss.

Another study found that participants consumed 35% fewer calories and lost an average of 7.7 pounds (3.5 kg) after alternating between 36 hours of fasting and 12 hours of unlimited eating over 4 weeks.

If you really want to maximize weight loss, adding an exercise regime to your life can help.

Research shows that combining alternate-day fasting with endurance exercise may cause twice as much weight loss than simply fasting.

A full fast every other day can be extreme, especially if you're new to fasting. Overeating on non-fasting days can also be tempting.

If you're new to intermittent fasting, ease into alternate-day fasting with a modified fasting plan.

Whether you start with a modified fasting plan or full fast, it's best to maintain a nutritious diet, incorporating high protein foods and low calorie vegetables to help you feel full.

The Warrior diet

The Warrior Diet is an intermittent fasting plan based on the eating patterns of ancient warriors.

Created in 2001 by Ori Hofmekler, the Warrior Diet is a bit more extreme than the 16:8 method but less restrictive than the Eat Fast Eat method.

It consists of eating very little for 20 hours during the day, and then eating as much food as desired throughout a 4-hour window at night.

The Warrior Diet encourages dieters to consume small amounts of dairy products, hard-boiled eggs, and raw fruits and vegetables, as well as non-calorie fluids during the 20-hour fast period.

After this 20-hour fast, people can essentially eat anything they want for a 4-hour window, but unprocessed, healthy, and organic foods are recommended.

While there's no research on the Warrior Diet specifically, human studies indicate that time-restricted feeding cycles can lead to weight loss

Time-restricted feeding cycles may have a variety of other health benefits. Studies show that time-restricted feeding cycles can prevent diabetes, slow tumor progression, delay aging, and increase lifespan in rodents.

More research is needed on the Warrior Diet to fully understand its benefits for weight loss.

The Warrior Diet may be difficult to follow, as it restricts substantial calorie consumption to just 4 hours per day. Overconsumption at night is a common challenge.

The Warrior Diet may also lead to disordered eating patterns. If you feel up for the challenge, talk to your doctor to see whether it's right for you.

SUMMARY

There are many varieties of intermittent fasting, each with their own benefits and challenges. Talk to your doctor to see which option may be right for you.

How intermittent fasting affects your hormones

Intermittent fasting may help you lose weight, but it can also affect your hormones.

That's because body fat is the body's way of storing energy (calories).

When you don't eat anything, your body makes several changes to make its stored energy more accessible.

Examples include changes in nervous system activity, as well as major changes in the levels of several crucial hormones.

Below are two metabolic changes that occur when you fast:

• Insulin. Insulin levels increase when you eat, and when you fast, they decrease dramatically. Lower levels of insulin facilitate fat burning.

• Norepinephrine (noradrenaline). Your nervous system sends norepinephrine to your fat cells, making them break down body fat into free fatty acids that can be burned for energy.

Interestingly, despite what some proponents of consuming 5–6 meals per day claim, short-term fasting may increase fat burning.

Research shows that alternate-day fasting trials lasting 3–12 weeks, as well as whole-day fasting trials lasting 12–24 weeks, reduce body weight and body fat .

Still, more research is needed to investigate the long-term effects of intermittent fasting.

Another hormone that's altered during a fast is human growth hormone (HGH), levels of which may increase as much as five-fold.

Previously, HGH was believed to help burn fat faster, but new research shows it may signal the brain to conserve energy, potentially making it harder to lose weight.

By activating a small population of agouti-related protein (AgRP) neurons, HGH may indirectly increase appetite and diminish energy metabolism.

SUMMARY

Short-term fasting leads to several bodily changes that promote fat burning. Nevertheless, skyrocketing HGH levels may indirectly decrease energy metabolism and combat continued weight loss.

Intermittent fasting helps you reduce calories and lose weight

The main reason that intermittent fasting works for weight loss is that it helps you eat fewer calories.

All of the different protocols involve skipping meals during the fasting periods.

Unless you compensate by eating much more during the eating periods, you'll be consuming fewer calories.

According to a 2014 review, intermittent fasting reduced body weight by 3–8% over a period of 3–24 weeks.

When examining the rate of weight loss, intermittent fasting may produce weight loss at a rate of approximately 0.55 to 1.65 pounds (0.25–0.75 kg) per week.

People also experienced a 4–7% reduction in waist circumference, indicating that they lost belly fat.

These results indicate that intermittent fasting can be a useful weight loss tool.

That said, the benefits of intermittent fasting go way beyond weight loss.

It also has numerous benefits for metabolic health, and it may even help reduce the risk of cardiovascular disease.

Although calorie counting is generally not required when doing intermittent fasting, the weight loss is mostly mediated by an overall reduction in calorie intake.

Studies comparing intermittent fasting and continuous calorie restriction show no difference in weight loss when calories are matched between groups.

SUMMARY

Intermittent fasting is a convenient way to lose weight without counting calories. Many studies show that it can help you lose weight and belly fat.

Intermittent fasting may help you maintain muscle mass when dieting

One of the worst side effects of dieting is that your body tends to lose muscle along with fat.

Interestingly, some studies have shown that intermittent fasting may be beneficial for maintaining muscle mass while losing body fat.

A scientific review found that intermittent calorie restriction caused a similar amount of weight loss as continuous calorie restriction — but with a much smaller reduction in muscle mass.

In the calorie restriction studies, 25% of the weight lost was muscle mass, compared with only 10% in the intermittent calorie restriction studies.

However, these studies had some limitations, so take the findings with a grain of salt. More recent studies haven't found any differences in lean mass or muscle mass with intermittent fasting when compared with other types of eating plans.

SUMMARY

While some evidence suggests that intermittent fasting, when compared with standard calorie restriction, could help you hold on to more muscle mass, more recent studies haven't supported the notion.

Intermittent fasting makes healthy eating simpler

For many, one of the main benefits of intermittent fasting is its simplicity.

Rather than counting calories, most intermittent fasting regimes simply require you to tell time.

The best dietary pattern for you is the one you can stick to in the long run. If intermittent fasting makes it easier for you to stick to a healthy diet, it will have obvious benefits for long-term health and weight maintenance.

SUMMARY

One of the main benefits of intermittent fasting is that it makes healthy eating simpler. This may make it easier to stick to a healthy diet in the long run.

How to succeed with an intermittent fasting protocol

There are several things you need to keep in mind if you want to lose weight with intermittent fasting:

1. Food quality. The foods you eat are still important. Try to eat mostly whole, single-ingredient foods.

2. Calories. Calories still count. Try to eat normally during the non-fasting periods, not so much that you compensate for the calories you missed when fasting.

3. Consistency. Just as with any other weight loss method, you need to stick with it for an extended period if you want it to work.

4. Patience. It can take your body some time to adapt to an intermittent

fasting protocol. Try to be consistent with your meal schedule, and it'll get easier.

Most of the popular intermittent fasting protocols also recommend exercise, such as strength training. This is very important if you want to burn mostly body fat while maintaining your muscle mass.

In the beginning, calorie counting is generally not required with intermittent fasting. However, if your weight loss stalls, calorie counting can be a useful tool.

SUMMARY

With intermittent fasting, you still need to eat healthy and maintain a calorie deficit if you want to lose weight. Being consistent is crucial, and exercise is important.

The bottom line

At the end of the day, intermittent fasting can be a useful weight loss tool.

Its related weight loss is primarily caused by a reduction in calorie intake, but some of its beneficial effects on hormones may also come into play.

While intermittent fasting is not for everyone, it may be highly beneficial for some people.